This Planner Belongs To;

_____

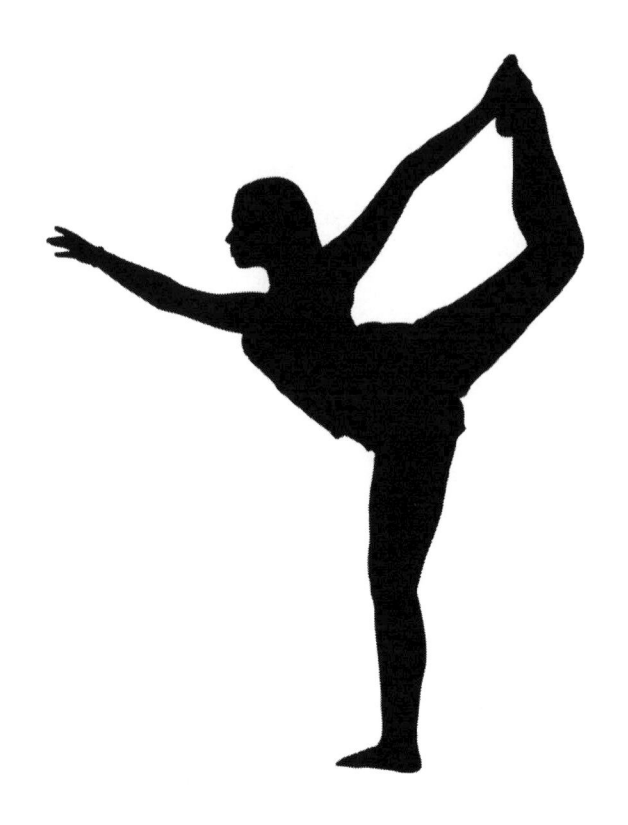

Want to maximize your results?
Download your Free Gift (instant download)
http://bit.ly/JOURNALFREEGIFT

© Copyright 2019 UltraLiving.com

ALL RIGHTS RESERVED

No part of this book may be reproduced or transmitted in any form whatsoever, electronic, or mechanical, including photocopying, recording, or by any informational storage or retrieval system without express written, dated and signed permission from the author.

Progress Tracker

Arm

Chest

Waist

Hips

Thigh

STARTING MEASUREMENTS:

WEIGHT:

LEFT ARM:

RIGHT ARM:

CHEST:

WAIST:

HIPS:

LEFT THIGH:

RIGHT THIGH:

My Journey

START DAY:
_____

PERSONAL GOALS:
_____
_____
_____

Healthy Breakfast Ideas

Healthy Breakfast Ideas

Healthy Lunch Ideas

Healthy Lunch Ideas

Healthy Dinner Ideas

Healthy Dinner Ideas

Healthy Snack Ideas

MY MISSION: TO BE SO BUSY LOVING MY LIFE THAT I HAVE NO TIME FOR HATE, REGRET, WORRY, FRET OR FEAR

Daily Wellness Tracker

Date: _____
S M T W T F S

Today's Fitness Focus

Cardio ☐ Strength ☐ Flexibility ☐ Rest ☐

Activity _____
_____

Duration: _____

Today I'm grateful for:

Energy Meter
1 > 2 > 3 > 4 > 5 > 6 > 7 > 8 > 9 > 10

Stress Indicator
Low   Ok   High

Water
☐ ☐ ☐ ☐ ☐ ☐ ☐ ☐

Fruits & Vegetables
☐ ☐ ☐ ☐ ☐ ☐ ☐

	Meal Tracker	Counter*
Breakfast		
Lunch		
Dinner		
Snacks		

* Calories, points, containers

Notes

THE BEGINNING IS ALWAYS TOUGH BUT ONCE I'M IN IT I BECOME UNSTOPPABLE

Daily Wellness Tracker

Date: _____
S M T W T F S

Today's Fitness Focus

Cardio ☐   Strength ☐   Flexibility ☐   Rest ☐

Activity _____
_____

Duration: _____

Today I'm grateful for:

Energy Meter
1 > 2 > 3 > 4 > 5 > 6 > 7 > 8 > 9 > 10

Stress Indicator
Low   Ok   High

Water
☐ ☐ ☐ ☐ ☐ ☐ ☐ ☐

Fruits & Vegetables
☐ ☐ ☐ ☐ ☐ ☐ ☐ ☐

	Meal Tracker	Counter*
Breakfast		
Lunch		
Dinner		
Snacks		

* Calories, points, containers

Notes

THIS IS NOT YOUR PRACTICE LIFE

TAKE TIME TO DO WHAT MAKES YOUR SOUL HAPPY

Daily Wellness Tracker

Date: _____
S M T W T F S

Today's Fitness Focus

Cardio ☐   Strength ☐   Flexibility ☐   Rest ☐

Activity _____
_____

Duration: _____

Today I'm grateful for:

Energy Meter

1 › 2 › 3 › 4 › 5 › 6 › 7 › 8 › 9 › 10 ›

Stress Indicator

Low   Ok   High

Water
☐ ☐ ☐ ☐ ☐ ☐ ☐ ☐

Fruits & Vegetables
☐ ☐ ☐ ☐ ☐ ☐ ☐

	Meal Tracker	Counter*
Breakfast		
Lunch		
Dinner		
Snacks		

* Calories, points, containers

Notes

START
where you are.
USE
what you have.
DO
what you can.

Daily Wellness Tracker

Date: _____
S M T W T F S

Today's Fitness Focus

Cardio Strength Flexibility Rest
☐   ☐   ☐   ☐

Activity _____
_____

Duration: _____

Today I'm grateful for:

Energy Meter

1 > 2 > 3 > 4 > 5 > 6 > 7 > 8 > 9 > 10

Stress Indicator

Low   Ok   High

Water
☐ ☐ ☐ ☐ ☐ ☐ ☐ ☐

Fruits & Vegetables
☐ ☐ ☐ ☐ ☐ ☐ ☐ ☐

	Meal Tracker	Counter*
Breakfast		
Lunch		
Dinner		
Snacks		

*Calories, points, containers

Notes

focus on how far you've come not how far you have to go

Daily Wellness Tracker

Date: _____
S M T W T F S

Today's Fitness Focus

Cardio ☐ Strength ☐ Flexibility ☐ Rest ☐

Activity _____
_____

Duration: _____

Today I'm grateful for:

Energy Meter

1 > 2 > 3 > 4 > 5 > 6 > 7 > 8 > 9 > 10 >

Stress Indicator

Low | Ok | High

Water
☐ ☐ ☐ ☐ ☐ ☐ ☐ ☐

Fruits & Vegetables
☐ ☐ ☐ ☐ ☐ ☐ ☐ ☐

	Meal Tracker	Counter*
Breakfast		
Lunch		
Dinner		
Snacks		

* Calories, points, containers

Notes

AND SO SHE DECIDED TO START LIVING THE LIFE SHE'D IMAGINED

Daily Wellness Tracker

Date: _____
S M T W T F S

Today's Fitness Focus

Cardio ☐   Strength ☐   Flexibility ☐   Rest ☐

Activity _____
_____

Duration: _____

Today I'm grateful for:

Energy Meter

1 > 2 > 3 > 4 > 5 > 6 > 7 > 8 > 9 > 10

Stress Indicator

Low   Ok   High

Water
☐ ☐ ☐ ☐ ☐ ☐ ☐ ☐

Fruits & Vegetables
☐ ☐ ☐ ☐ ☐ ☐ ☐

	Meal Tracker	Counter*
Breakfast		
Lunch		
Dinner		
Snacks		

*Calories, points, containers

Notes

You're always one decision away from a totally different life

Daily Wellness Tracker

Date: _____
S M T W T F S

Today's Fitness Focus

Cardio ☐ Strength ☐ Flexibility ☐ Rest ☐

Activity _____
_____

Duration: _____

Today I'm grateful for:

Energy Meter
1 > 2 > 3 > 4 > 5 > 6 > 7 > 8 > 9 > 10 >

Stress Indicator
Low | Ok | High

Water
☐ ☐ ☐ ☐ ☐ ☐ ☐ ☐

Fruits & Vegetables
☐ ☐ ☐ ☐ ☐ ☐ ☐ ☐

	Meal Tracker	Counter*
Breakfast		
Lunch		
Dinner		
Snacks		

* Calories, points, containers

Notes

Don't forget that you're human. It's okay to have a meltdown. Just don't unpack and live there. Cry it out and then refocus on where you are headed.

Daily Wellness Tracker

Date: _____
S M T W T F S

Today's Fitness Focus

Cardio ☐   Strength ☐   Flexibility ☐   Rest ☐

Activity _____
_____

Duration: _____

Today I'm grateful for:

Energy Meter

1 > 2 > 3 > 4 > 5 > 6 > 7 > 8 > 9 > 10 >

Stress Indicator

Low   Ok   High

Water
☐ ☐ ☐ ☐ ☐ ☐ ☐ ☐

Fruits & Vegetables
☐ ☐ ☐ ☐ ☐ ☐ ☐ ☐

	Meal Tracker	Counter*
Breakfast		
Lunch		
Dinner		
Snacks		

* Calories, points, containers

Notes

Be the girl who decided to go for it

Daily Wellness Tracker

Date: _____
S M T W T F S

Today's Fitness Focus

Cardio ☐   Strength ☐   Flexibility ☐   Rest ☐

Activity _____
_____

Duration: _____

Today I'm grateful for:

Energy Meter

1 › 2 › 3 › 4 › 5 › 6 › 7 › 8 › 9 › 10 ›

Stress Indicator

Low ⬇   Ok   High ⬆

Water
☐ ☐ ☐ ☐ ☐ ☐ ☐ ☐

Fruits & Vegetables
☐ ☐ ☐ ☐ ☐ ☐ ☐ ☐

	Meal Tracker	Counter*
Breakfast		
Lunch		
Dinner		
Snacks		

* Calories, points, containers

Notes

Exercise is a celebration of what your body can do not a punishment for what you ate

Daily Wellness Tracker

Date: _____
S M T W T F S

Today's Fitness Focus

Cardio Strength Flexibility Rest
☐   ☐   ☐   ☐

Activity _____
_____

Duration: _____

Today I'm grateful for:

Energy Meter

1 > 2 > 3 > 4 > 5 > 6 > 7 > 8 > 9 > 10

Stress Indicator

Low   Ok   High

Water
☐ ☐ ☐ ☐ ☐ ☐ ☐ ☐

Fruits & Vegetables
☐ ☐ ☐ ☐ ☐ ☐ ☐

	Meal Tracker	Counter*
Breakfast		
Lunch		
Dinner		
Snacks		

* Calories, points, containers

Notes

I didn't come this far to only come this far

Daily Wellness Tracker

Date: _____
S M T W T F S

Today's Fitness Focus

Cardio ☐ Strength ☐ Flexibility ☐ Rest ☐

Activity _____

_____

Duration: _____

Today I'm grateful for:

Energy Meter

1 > 2 > 3 > 4 > 5 > 6 > 7 > 8 > 9 > 10

Stress Indicator

Low   Ok   High

Water

☐ ☐ ☐ ☐ ☐ ☐ ☐ ☐

Fruits & Vegetables

☐ ☐ ☐ ☐ ☐ ☐ ☐

	Meal Tracker	Counter*
Breakfast		
Lunch		
Dinner		
Snacks		

* Calories, points, containers

Notes

Don't be in such a rush to figure everything out. **Embrace the unknown** and let your life surprise you.

Daily Wellness Tracker

Date: _____
S M T W T F S

Today's Fitness Focus

Cardio ☐ Strength ☐ Flexibility ☐ Rest ☐

Activity _____

_____

Duration: _____

Today I'm grateful for:

Energy Meter

1 > 2 > 3 > 4 > 5 > 6 > 7 > 8 > 9 > 10

Stress Indicator

Low ⬇ Ok High ⬆

Water
☐ ☐ ☐ ☐ ☐ ☐ ☐ ☐

Fruits & Vegetables
☐ ☐ ☐ ☐ ☐ ☐ ☐

	Meal Tracker	Counter*
Breakfast		
Lunch		
Dinner		
Snacks		

*Calories, points, containers

Notes

Today I will love myself enough to exercise

Daily Wellness Tracker

Date: _____
S M T W T F S

Today's Fitness Focus

Cardio ☐   Strength ☐   Flexibility ☐   Rest ☐

Activity _____
_____

Duration: _____

Today I'm grateful for:

Energy Meter
1 > 2 > 3 > 4 > 5 > 6 > 7 > 8 > 9 > 10 >

Stress Indicator
Low   Ok   High

Water
☐ ☐ ☐ ☐ ☐ ☐ ☐ ☐

Fruits & Vegetables
☐ ☐ ☐ ☐ ☐ ☐ ☐ ☐

	Meal Tracker	Counter*
Breakfast		
Lunch		
Dinner		
Snacks		

* Calories, points, containers

Notes

When women support each other, incredible things happen

Daily Wellness Tracker

Date: _____
S M T W T F S

Today's Fitness Focus

- [ ] Cardio
- [ ] Strength
- [ ] Flexibility
- [ ] Rest

Activity _____

_____

Duration: _____

Energy Meter

1 › 2 › 3 › 4 › 5 › 6 › 7 › 8 › 9 › 10 ›

Stress Indicator

Low · Ok · High

Today I'm grateful for:

Water
☐ ☐ ☐ ☐ ☐ ☐ ☐ ☐

Fruits & Vegetables
☐ ☐ ☐ ☐ ☐ ☐ ☐

	Meal Tracker	Counter*
Breakfast		
Lunch		
Dinner		
Snacks		

* Calories, points, containers

Notes

Accomplishments

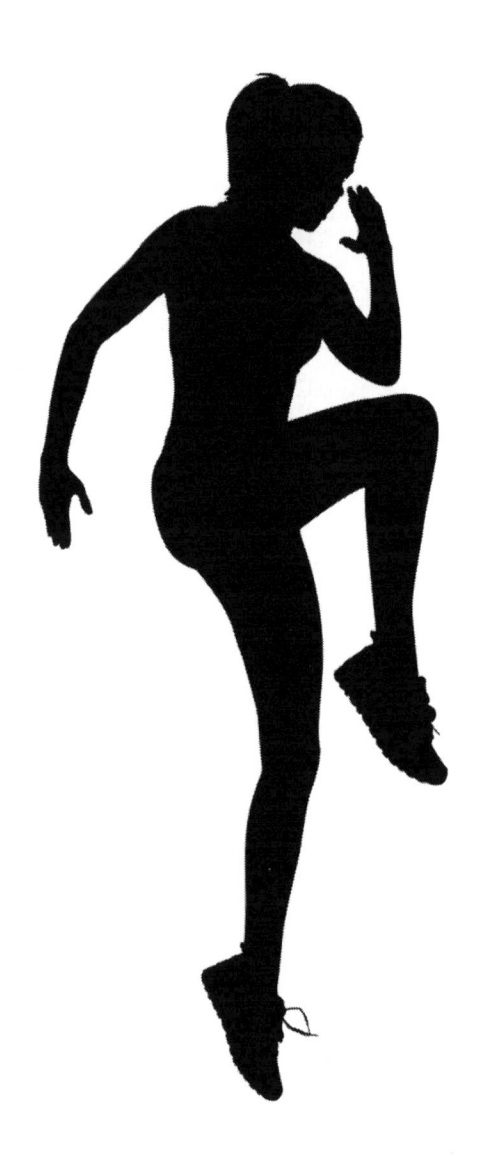

START WEIGHT:

CURRENT WEIGHT:

TOTAL LOSS:

I can do anything...

MY ACCOMPLISHMENTS:

NOTES TO SELF:

Believe in Yourself

Daily Wellness Tracker

Date: _____
S M T W T F S

Today's Fitness Focus

Cardio ☐   Strength ☐   Flexibility ☐   Rest ☐

Activity _____
_____

Duration: _____

Today I'm grateful for:

Energy Meter
1 › 2 › 3 › 4 › 5 › 6 › 7 › 8 › 9 › 10

Stress Indicator
Low   Ok   High

Water
☐ ☐ ☐ ☐ ☐ ☐ ☐ ☐

Fruits & Vegetables
☐ ☐ ☐ ☐ ☐ ☐ ☐

	Meal Tracker	Counter*
Breakfast		
Lunch		
Dinner		
Snacks		

*Calories, points, containers

Notes

Trust the wait

Embrace the uncertainty

Enjoy the beauty of becoming

When nothing is certain,

anything is possible

Daily Wellness Tracker

Date: _____
S M T W T F S

Today's Fitness Focus

Cardio ☐ Strength ☐ Flexibility ☐ Rest ☐

Activity _____
_____

Duration: _____

Today I'm grateful for:

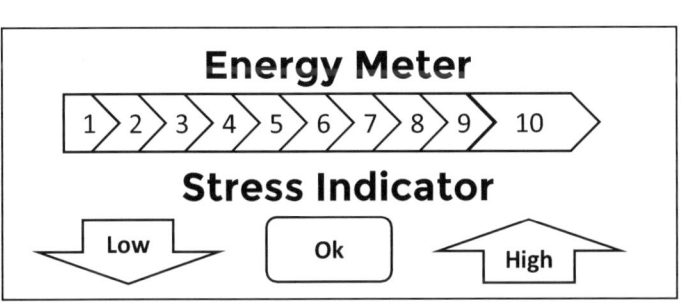

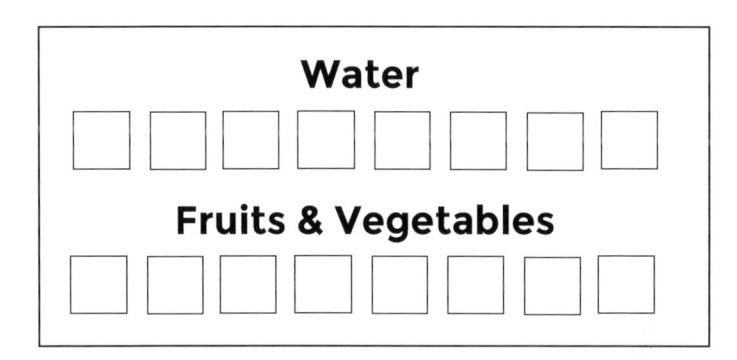

Energy Meter
1 > 2 > 3 > 4 > 5 > 6 > 7 > 8 > 9 > 10

Stress Indicator
Low   Ok   High

Water
☐ ☐ ☐ ☐ ☐ ☐ ☐ ☐

Fruits & Vegetables
☐ ☐ ☐ ☐ ☐ ☐ ☐

	Meal Tracker	Counter*
Breakfast		
Lunch		
Dinner		
Snacks		

* Calories, points, containers

Notes

You've got a new story to write. And it looks nothing like your past.

Daily Wellness Tracker

Date: _____
S M T W T F S

Today's Fitness Focus

Cardio ☐ Strength ☐ Flexibility ☐ Rest ☐

Activity _____

_____

Duration: _____

Today I'm grateful for:

Energy Meter

1 > 2 > 3 > 4 > 5 > 6 > 7 > 8 > 9 > 10

Stress Indicator

Low | Ok | High

Water
☐ ☐ ☐ ☐ ☐ ☐ ☐ ☐

Fruits & Vegetables
☐ ☐ ☐ ☐ ☐ ☐ ☐

	Meal Tracker	Counter*
Breakfast		
Lunch		
Dinner		
Snacks		

* Calories, points, containers

Notes

Stay patient and trust your journey

Daily Wellness Tracker

Date: _____
S M T W T F S

Today's Fitness Focus

Cardio Strength Flexibility Rest
☐   ☐   ☐   ☐

Activity _____

_____

Duration: _____

Today I'm grateful for:

Energy Meter

1 > 2 > 3 > 4 > 5 > 6 > 7 > 8 > 9 > 10

Stress Indicator

Low   Ok   High

Water
☐ ☐ ☐ ☐ ☐ ☐ ☐ ☐

Fruits & Vegetables
☐ ☐ ☐ ☐ ☐ ☐ ☐

Meal Tracker | Counter*

	Meal Tracker	Counter*
Breakfast		
Lunch		
Dinner		
Snacks		

* Calories, points, containers

Notes

I want to inspire people... I want someone to look at me and say Because of you I didn't give up.

Daily Wellness Tracker

Date: _____
S M T W T F S

Today's Fitness Focus

Cardio ☐ Strength ☐ Flexibility ☐ Rest ☐

Activity _____
_____

Duration: _____

Today I'm grateful for:

Energy Meter
1 > 2 > 3 > 4 > 5 > 6 > 7 > 8 > 9 > 10

Stress Indicator
Low | Ok | High

Water
☐ ☐ ☐ ☐ ☐ ☐ ☐ ☐

Fruits & Vegetables
☐ ☐ ☐ ☐ ☐ ☐ ☐

	Meal Tracker	Counter*
Breakfast		
Lunch		
Dinner		
Snacks		

* Calories, points, containers

Notes

I'm blessed

with everything I need. I am working hard towards everything I want. And most of all I appreciate & Thank God for what I have.

Daily Wellness Tracker

Date: _____
S M T W T F S

Today's Fitness Focus

Cardio ☐ Strength ☐ Flexibility ☐ Rest ☐

Activity _____
_____

Duration: _____

Energy Meter

1 > 2 > 3 > 4 > 5 > 6 > 7 > 8 > 9 > 10

Stress Indicator

Low | Ok | High

Today I'm grateful for:

Water
☐ ☐ ☐ ☐ ☐ ☐ ☐ ☐

Fruits & Vegetables
☐ ☐ ☐ ☐ ☐ ☐ ☐

	Meal Tracker	Counter*
Breakfast		
Lunch		
Dinner		
Snacks		

* Calories, points, containers

Notes

Eat healthy, workout, read books, be positive, expand your consciousness. Do things that will help you become a better person inside and out.

Daily Wellness Tracker

Date: _____
S M T W T F S

Today's Fitness Focus

Cardio ☐   Strength ☐   Flexibility ☐   Rest ☐

Activity _____
_____

Duration: _____

Today I'm grateful for:

Energy Meter
1 > 2 > 3 > 4 > 5 > 6 > 7 > 8 > 9 > 10 >

Stress Indicator
Low   Ok   High

Water
☐ ☐ ☐ ☐ ☐ ☐ ☐ ☐

Fruits & Vegetables
☐ ☐ ☐ ☐ ☐ ☐ ☐ ☐

	Meal Tracker	Counter*
Breakfast		
Lunch		
Dinner		
Snacks		

*Calories, points, containers

Notes

If you want to change your life, begin by changing your words. Start speaking the words of your dreams, of who you want to become, not the words of fear and failure
– Robert Kiyosaki

Daily Wellness Tracker

Date: _____
S M T W T F S

Today's Fitness Focus

Cardio ☐   Strength ☐   Flexibility ☐   Rest ☐

Activity _____

_____

Duration: _____

Today I'm grateful for:

Energy Meter

1 > 2 > 3 > 4 > 5 > 6 > 7 > 8 > 9 > 10

Stress Indicator

Low   Ok   High

Water
☐ ☐ ☐ ☐ ☐ ☐ ☐ ☐

Fruits & Vegetables
☐ ☐ ☐ ☐ ☐ ☐ ☐

	Meal Tracker	Counter*
Breakfast		
Lunch		
Dinner		
Snacks		

* Calories, points, containers

Notes

Discipline is doing what needs to be done even if you don't want to do it.

Daily Wellness Tracker

Date: _____
S M T W T F S

Today's Fitness Focus

Cardio Strength Flexibility Rest
☐   ☐   ☐   ☐

Activity _____
_____

Duration: _____

Today I'm grateful for:

Energy Meter

1 > 2 > 3 > 4 > 5 > 6 > 7 > 8 > 9 > 10

Stress Indicator

Low   Ok   High

Water
☐ ☐ ☐ ☐ ☐ ☐ ☐ ☐

Fruits & Vegetables
☐ ☐ ☐ ☐ ☐ ☐ ☐

	Meal Tracker	Counter*
Breakfast		
Lunch		
Dinner		
Snacks		

*Calories, points, containers

Notes

And Suddenly You Just Know It's Time To start Something New & Trust The

Magic Of Beginnings

Daily Wellness Tracker

Date: _____
S M T W T F S

Today's Fitness Focus

Cardio ☐   Strength ☐   Flexibility ☐   Rest ☐

Activity _____
_____

Duration: _____

Today I'm grateful for:

Energy Meter
1 > 2 > 3 > 4 > 5 > 6 > 7 > 8 > 9 > 10

Stress Indicator
Low   Ok   High

Water
☐ ☐ ☐ ☐ ☐ ☐ ☐ ☐

Fruits & Vegetables
☐ ☐ ☐ ☐ ☐ ☐ ☐ ☐

	Meal Tracker	Counter*
Breakfast		
Lunch		
Dinner		
Snacks		

* Calories, points, containers

Notes

To Be Worthy Does Not Mean To Be Perfect

Daily Wellness Tracker

Date: _____
S M T W T F S

Today's Fitness Focus

Cardio Strength Flexibility Rest
☐   ☐   ☐   ☐

Activity _____
_____

Duration: _____

Today I'm grateful for:

Energy Meter
1 > 2 > 3 > 4 > 5 > 6 > 7 > 8 > 9 > 10

Stress Indicator
Low   Ok   High

Water
☐ ☐ ☐ ☐ ☐ ☐ ☐ ☐

Fruits & Vegetables
☐ ☐ ☐ ☐ ☐ ☐ ☐ ☐

	Meal Tracker	Counter*
Breakfast		
Lunch		
Dinner		
Snacks		

* Calories, points, containers

Notes

Know That You Can Start Late, Look Different, Be Uncertain And Still SUCCEED

Daily Wellness Tracker

Date: _____
S M T W T F S

Today's Fitness Focus

Cardio Strength Flexibility Rest
☐   ☐   ☐   ☐

Activity _____
_____

Duration: _____

Today I'm grateful for:

Energy Meter

1 > 2 > 3 > 4 > 5 > 6 > 7 > 8 > 9 > 10

Stress Indicator

Low   Ok   High

Water
☐ ☐ ☐ ☐ ☐ ☐ ☐ ☐

Fruits & Vegetables
☐ ☐ ☐ ☐ ☐ ☐ ☐

	Meal Tracker	Counter*
Breakfast		
Lunch		
Dinner		
Snacks		

* Calories, points, containers

Notes

I've always loved butterflies because they remind us that it's never too late to transform ourselves.

— Drew Barrymore

Daily Wellness Tracker

Date: _____
S M T W T F S

Today's Fitness Focus

Cardio ☐   Strength ☐   Flexibility ☐   Rest ☐

Activity _____
_____

Duration: _____

Today I'm grateful for:

Energy Meter
1 > 2 > 3 > 4 > 5 > 6 > 7 > 8 > 9 > 10

Stress Indicator
Low   Ok   High

Water
☐ ☐ ☐ ☐ ☐ ☐ ☐ ☐

Fruits & Vegetables
☐ ☐ ☐ ☐ ☐ ☐ ☐ ☐

	Meal Tracker	Counter*
Breakfast		
Lunch		
Dinner		
Snacks		

* Calories, points, containers

Notes

You can't go back and change the beginning, but you can start where you are and change the ending

— C.S. Lewis

Daily Wellness Tracker

Date: _____
S M T W T F S

Today's Fitness Focus

Cardio ☐ Strength ☐ Flexibility ☐ Rest ☐

Activity _____
_____

Duration: _____

Today I'm grateful for:

Energy Meter
1 > 2 > 3 > 4 > 5 > 6 > 7 > 8 > 9 > 10

Stress Indicator
Low | Ok | High

Water
☐ ☐ ☐ ☐ ☐ ☐ ☐ ☐

Fruits & Vegetables
☐ ☐ ☐ ☐ ☐ ☐ ☐

	Meal Tracker	Counter*
Breakfast		
Lunch		
Dinner		
Snacks		

* Calories, points, containers

Notes

Accomplishments

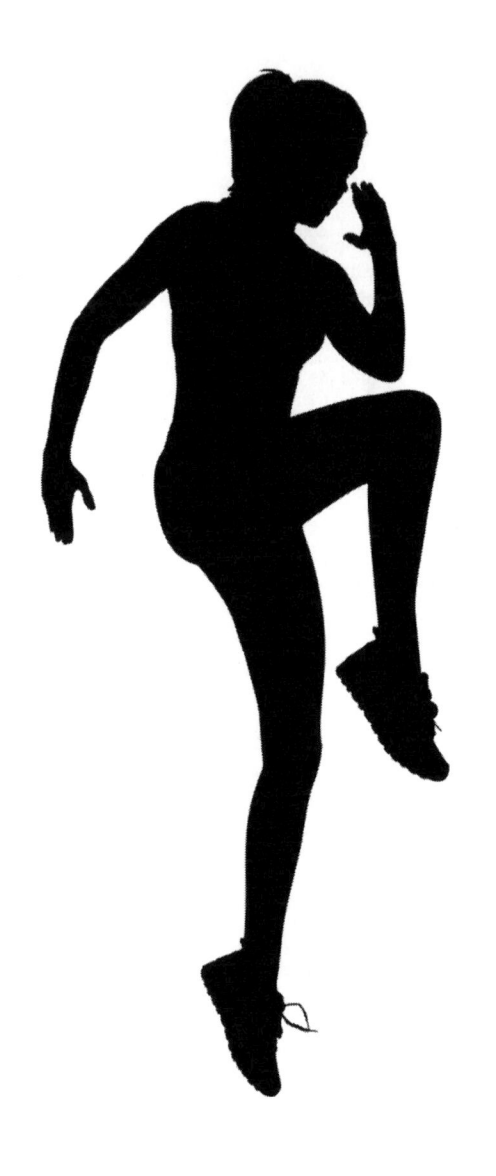

START WEIGHT:

CURRENT WEIGHT:

TOTAL LOSS:

I can do anything...

MY ACCOMPLISHMENTS:

NOTES TO SELF:

Believe in Yourself

Daily Wellness Tracker

Date: _____
S M T W T F S

Today's Fitness Focus

Cardio ☐   Strength ☐   Flexibility ☐   Rest ☐

Activity _____

_____

Duration: _____

Today I'm grateful for:

Energy Meter

1 › 2 › 3 › 4 › 5 › 6 › 7 › 8 › 9 › 10

Stress Indicator

Low   Ok   High

Water
☐ ☐ ☐ ☐ ☐ ☐ ☐ ☐

Fruits & Vegetables
☐ ☐ ☐ ☐ ☐ ☐ ☐

	Meal Tracker	Counter*
Breakfast		
Lunch		
Dinner		
Snacks		

* Calories, points, containers

Notes

In Two Weeks, You'll Feel It. In Four Weeks, You'll See It. In Eight Weeks, You'll Hear It.

Daily Wellness Tracker

Date: _____
S M T W T F S

Today's Fitness Focus

Cardio ☐ Strength ☐ Flexibility ☐ Rest ☐

Activity: _____
_____

Duration: _____

Today I'm grateful for:

Energy Meter
1 › 2 › 3 › 4 › 5 › 6 › 7 › 8 › 9 › 10

Stress Indicator
Low | Ok | High

Water
☐ ☐ ☐ ☐ ☐ ☐ ☐ ☐

Fruits & Vegetables
☐ ☐ ☐ ☐ ☐ ☐ ☐

	Meal Tracker	Counter*
Breakfast		
Lunch		
Dinner		
Snacks		

* Calories, points, containers

Notes

The best part about life? Every morning you have a new opportunity to become a happier version of yourself.

Daily Wellness Tracker

Date: _____
S M T W T F S

Today's Fitness Focus

Cardio Strength Flexibility Rest
☐   ☐   ☐   ☐

Activity _____
_____

Duration: _____

Today I'm grateful for:

Energy Meter

1 > 2 > 3 > 4 > 5 > 6 > 7 > 8 > 9 > 10

Stress Indicator

Low   Ok   High

Water
☐ ☐ ☐ ☐ ☐ ☐ ☐ ☐

Fruits & Vegetables
☐ ☐ ☐ ☐ ☐ ☐ ☐

	Meal Tracker	Counter*
Breakfast		
Lunch		
Dinner		
Snacks		

*Calories, points, containers

Notes

...and she just knew that EVERYTHING would work out... It Always does.

Daily Wellness Tracker

Date: _____
S M T W T F S

Today's Fitness Focus

Cardio ☐   Strength ☐   Flexibility ☐   Rest ☐

Activity _____

_____

Duration: _____

Today I'm grateful for:

Energy Meter
1 > 2 > 3 > 4 > 5 > 6 > 7 > 8 > 9 > 10

Stress Indicator
Low   Ok   High

Water
☐ ☐ ☐ ☐ ☐ ☐ ☐ ☐

Fruits & Vegetables
☐ ☐ ☐ ☐ ☐ ☐ ☐

	Meal Tracker	Counter*
Breakfast		
Lunch		
Dinner		
Snacks		

* Calories, points, containers

Notes

When you can't control whats happening, challenge yourself to control the way you respond to whats happening. That's where your power is.

Daily Wellness Tracker

Date: _____
S M T W T F S

Today's Fitness Focus

Cardio ☐   Strength ☐   Flexibility ☐   Rest ☐

Activity _____
_____

Duration: _____

Today I'm grateful for:

Energy Meter
1 > 2 > 3 > 4 > 5 > 6 > 7 > 8 > 9 > 10

Stress Indicator
Low ⬇   Ok   High ⬆

Water
☐ ☐ ☐ ☐ ☐ ☐ ☐ ☐

Fruits & Vegetables
☐ ☐ ☐ ☐ ☐ ☐ ☐

	Meal Tracker	Counter*
Breakfast		
Lunch		
Dinner		
Snacks		

*Calories, points, containers

Notes

Sometimes you need to step outside, get some fresh air, & remind yourself of who you are & who you want to be.

Daily Wellness Tracker

Date: _____
S M T W T F S

Today's Fitness Focus

Cardio ☐   Strength ☐   Flexibility ☐   Rest ☐

Activity _____
_____

Duration: _____

Energy Meter

1 > 2 > 3 > 4 > 5 > 6 > 7 > 8 > 9 > 10

Stress Indicator

Low   Ok   High

Today I'm grateful for:

Water
☐ ☐ ☐ ☐ ☐ ☐ ☐ ☐

Fruits & Vegetables
☐ ☐ ☐ ☐ ☐ ☐ ☐

	Meal Tracker	Counter*
Breakfast		
Lunch		
Dinner		
Snacks		

*Calories, points, containers

Notes

Live Every Day With INTENTION

Daily Wellness Tracker

Date: _____
S M T W T F S

Today's Fitness Focus

Cardio ☐ Strength ☐ Flexibility ☐ Rest ☐

Activity _____
_____

Duration: _____

Today I'm grateful for:

Energy Meter
1 > 2 > 3 > 4 > 5 > 6 > 7 > 8 > 9 > 10

Stress Indicator
Low | Ok | High

Water
☐ ☐ ☐ ☐ ☐ ☐ ☐ ☐

Fruits & Vegetables
☐ ☐ ☐ ☐ ☐ ☐ ☐ ☐

	Meal Tracker	Counter*
Breakfast		
Lunch		
Dinner		
Snacks		

*Calories, points, containers

Notes

if you get Tired, learn to REST, Not To Quit

Daily Wellness Tracker

Date: _____
S M T W T F S

Today's Fitness Focus

Cardio ☐ Strength ☐ Flexibility ☐ Rest ☐

Activity _____
_____

Duration: _____

Today I'm grateful for:

Energy Meter
1 > 2 > 3 > 4 > 5 > 6 > 7 > 8 > 9 > 10

Stress Indicator
Low | Ok | High

Water
☐ ☐ ☐ ☐ ☐ ☐ ☐ ☐

Fruits & Vegetables
☐ ☐ ☐ ☐ ☐ ☐ ☐ ☐

	Meal Tracker	Counter*
Breakfast		
Lunch		
Dinner		
Snacks		

*Calories, points, containers

Notes

Note to self:
All you have to do is show up.
Be late.
Be scared.
Be a mess.
Be weird.
Be confused.
Just BE there.
You'll figure out the rest as you go.
- Nanea Hoffman

Daily Wellness Tracker

Date: _____
S M T W T F S

Today's Fitness Focus

Cardio Strength Flexibility Rest
☐   ☐   ☐   ☐

Activity _____
_____

Duration: _____

Today I'm grateful for:

Energy Meter

1 > 2 > 3 > 4 > 5 > 6 > 7 > 8 > 9 > 10

Stress Indicator

Low   Ok   High

Water
☐ ☐ ☐ ☐ ☐ ☐ ☐ ☐

Fruits & Vegetables
☐ ☐ ☐ ☐ ☐ ☐ ☐

	Meal Tracker	Counter*
Breakfast		
Lunch		
Dinner		
Snacks		

* Calories, points, containers

Notes

The best view comes after the hardest climb

Daily Wellness Tracker

Date: _____
S M T W T F S

Today's Fitness Focus

Cardio ☐   Strength ☐   Flexibility ☐   Rest ☐

Activity _____
_____

Duration: _____

Today I'm grateful for:

Energy Meter
1 > 2 > 3 > 4 > 5 > 6 > 7 > 8 > 9 > 10

Stress Indicator
Low ↓   Ok   High ↑

Water
☐ ☐ ☐ ☐ ☐ ☐ ☐ ☐

Fruits & Vegetables
☐ ☐ ☐ ☐ ☐ ☐ ☐

	Meal Tracker	Counter*
Breakfast		
Lunch		
Dinner		
Snacks		

*Calories, points, containers

Notes

Courage doesn't always roar. Sometimes courage is the quiet voice at the end of the day saying I will try again tomorrow.

- Mary Anne Radmacher

Daily Wellness Tracker

Date: _____
S M T W T F S

Today's Fitness Focus

Cardio Strength Flexibility Rest
☐　　　☐　　　　☐　　　　☐

Activity _____
_____

Duration: _____

Today I'm grateful for:

Energy Meter
1 2 3 4 5 6 7 8 9 10

Stress Indicator
Low   Ok   High

Water
☐ ☐ ☐ ☐ ☐ ☐ ☐ ☐

Fruits & Vegetables
☐ ☐ ☐ ☐ ☐ ☐ ☐

	Meal Tracker	Counter*
Breakfast		
Lunch		
Dinner		
Snacks		

* Calories, points, containers

Notes

Accept what is, let go of what was, and have faith in what will be.

Daily Wellness Tracker

Date: _____
S M T W T F S

Today's Fitness Focus

Cardio ☐ Strength ☐ Flexibility ☐ Rest ☐

Activity _____
_____

Duration: _____

Today I'm grateful for:

Energy Meter
1 > 2 > 3 > 4 > 5 > 6 > 7 > 8 > 9 > 10

Stress Indicator
Low   Ok   High

Water
☐ ☐ ☐ ☐ ☐ ☐ ☐ ☐

Fruits & Vegetables
☐ ☐ ☐ ☐ ☐ ☐ ☐

	Meal Tracker	Counter*
Breakfast		
Lunch		
Dinner		
Snacks		

*Calories, points, containers

Notes

Your relationship with yourself sets the tone for every other relationship you have.

Daily Wellness Tracker

Date: _____
S M T W T F S

Today's Fitness Focus

Cardio ☐   Strength ☐   Flexibility ☐   Rest ☐

Activity _____
_____

Duration: _____

Today I'm grateful for:

Energy Meter
1 › 2 › 3 › 4 › 5 › 6 › 7 › 8 › 9 › 10

Stress Indicator
Low   Ok   High

Water
☐ ☐ ☐ ☐ ☐ ☐ ☐ ☐

Fruits & Vegetables
☐ ☐ ☐ ☐ ☐ ☐ ☐

	Meal Tracker	Counter*
Breakfast		
Lunch		
Dinner		
Snacks		

*Calories, points, containers

Notes

Results happen over time, not overnight. Work hard, stay consistent and be patient.

Daily Wellness Tracker

Date: _____
S M T W T F S

Today's Fitness Focus

Cardio ☐   Strength ☐   Flexibility ☐   Rest ☐

Activity _____
_____

Duration: _____

Energy Meter

1 > 2 > 3 > 4 > 5 > 6 > 7 > 8 > 9 > 10

Stress Indicator

Low   Ok   High

Today I'm grateful for:

Water
☐ ☐ ☐ ☐ ☐ ☐ ☐ ☐

Fruits & Vegetables
☐ ☐ ☐ ☐ ☐ ☐ ☐ ☐

	Meal Tracker	Counter*
Breakfast		
Lunch		
Dinner		
Snacks		

* Calories, points, containers

Notes

Accomplishments

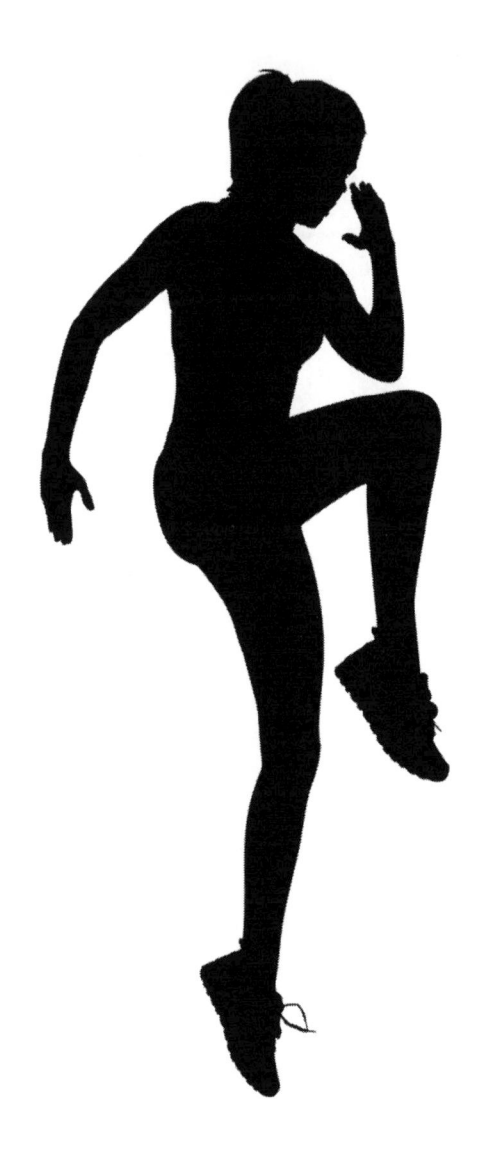

START WEIGHT:

CURRENT WEIGHT:

TOTAL LOSS:

I can do anything...

MY ACCOMPLISHMENTS:

NOTES TO SELF:

Believe in Yourself

Daily Wellness Tracker

Date: _____
S M T W T F S

Today's Fitness Focus

Cardio ☐ Strength ☐ Flexibility ☐ Rest ☐

Activity _____
_____

Duration: _____

Today I'm grateful for:

Energy Meter
1 > 2 > 3 > 4 > 5 > 6 > 7 > 8 > 9 > 10

Stress Indicator
Low   Ok   High

Water
☐ ☐ ☐ ☐ ☐ ☐ ☐ ☐

Fruits & Vegetables
☐ ☐ ☐ ☐ ☐ ☐ ☐

	Meal Tracker	Counter*
Breakfast		
Lunch		
Dinner		
Snacks		

* Calories, points, containers

Notes

Don't just be good to others be good to yourself too.

Daily Wellness Tracker

Date: _____
S M T W T F S

Today's Fitness Focus

Cardio ☐   Strength ☐   Flexibility ☐   Rest ☐

Activity _____
_____

Duration: _____

Today I'm grateful for:

Energy Meter

1 2 3 4 5 6 7 8 9 10

Stress Indicator

Low   Ok   High

Water
☐ ☐ ☐ ☐ ☐ ☐ ☐ ☐

Fruits & Vegetables
☐ ☐ ☐ ☐ ☐ ☐ ☐

	Meal Tracker	Counter*
Breakfast		
Lunch		
Dinner		
Snacks		

*Calories, points, containers

Notes

It's going to take some time but I will become the best version of ME.

Daily Wellness Tracker

Date: _____
S M T W T F S

Today's Fitness Focus

Cardio ☐   Strength ☐   Flexibility ☐   Rest ☐

Activity _____
_____

Duration: _____

Today I'm grateful for:

Energy Meter
1 › 2 › 3 › 4 › 5 › 6 › 7 › 8 › 9 › 10

Stress Indicator
Low   Ok   High

Water
☐ ☐ ☐ ☐ ☐ ☐ ☐ ☐

Fruits & Vegetables
☐ ☐ ☐ ☐ ☐ ☐ ☐

	Meal Tracker	Counter*
Breakfast		
Lunch		
Dinner		
Snacks		

*Calories, points, containers

Notes

It is a shame for a women to grow old without ever seeing the strength and beauty of which her body is capable.

Daily Wellness Tracker

Date: _____
S M T W T F S

Today's Fitness Focus

Cardio ☐ Strength ☐ Flexibility ☐ Rest ☐

Activity _____
_____

Duration: _____

Today I'm grateful for:

Energy Meter
1 > 2 > 3 > 4 > 5 > 6 > 7 > 8 > 9 > 10

Stress Indicator
Low   Ok   High

Water
☐ ☐ ☐ ☐ ☐ ☐ ☐ ☐

Fruits & Vegetables
☐ ☐ ☐ ☐ ☐ ☐ ☐ ☐

	Meal Tracker	Counter*
Breakfast		
Lunch		
Dinner		
Snacks		

* Calories, points, containers

Notes

You have to fight through some bad days to earn the best days of your life.

Daily Wellness Tracker

Date: _____
S M T W T F S

Today's Fitness Focus

Cardio Strength Flexibility Rest
☐   ☐   ☐   ☐

Activity _____

_____

Duration: _____

Today I'm grateful for:

Energy Meter
1 > 2 > 3 > 4 > 5 > 6 > 7 > 8 > 9 > 10

Stress Indicator
Low   Ok   High

Water
☐ ☐ ☐ ☐ ☐ ☐ ☐ ☐

Fruits & Vegetables
☐ ☐ ☐ ☐ ☐ ☐ ☐ ☐

	Meal Tracker	Counter*
Breakfast		
Lunch		
Dinner		
Snacks		

*Calories, points, containers

Notes

You Are Strong Enough & You Will Succeed

Daily Wellness Tracker

Date: _____
S M T W T F S

Today's Fitness Focus

Cardio ☐   Strength ☐   Flexibility ☐   Rest ☐

Activity _____
_____

Duration: _____

Today I'm grateful for:

Energy Meter

1 > 2 > 3 > 4 > 5 > 6 > 7 > 8 > 9 > 10

Stress Indicator

Low   Ok   High

Water
☐ ☐ ☐ ☐ ☐ ☐ ☐ ☐

Fruits & Vegetables
☐ ☐ ☐ ☐ ☐ ☐ ☐

Meal Tracker | Counter*

	Meal Tracker	Counter*
Breakfast		
Lunch		
Dinner		
Snacks		

*Calories, points, containers

Notes

SOMETIMES THE BRAVEST AND MOST IMPORTANT THING YOU CAN DO IS JUST SHOW UP

Daily Wellness Tracker

Date: _____
S M T W T F S

Today's Fitness Focus

Cardio ☐   Strength ☐   Flexibility ☐   Rest ☐

Activity _____

_____

Duration: _____

Energy Meter

1 › 2 › 3 › 4 › 5 › 6 › 7 › 8 › 9 › 10

Stress Indicator

Low   Ok   High

Today I'm grateful for:

Water
☐ ☐ ☐ ☐ ☐ ☐ ☐ ☐

Fruits & Vegetables
☐ ☐ ☐ ☐ ☐ ☐ ☐

	Meal Tracker	Counter*
Breakfast		
Lunch		
Dinner		
Snacks		

* Calories, points, containers

Notes

Sometimes the smallest step in the right direction ends up being the biggest step of your life. Tip toe if you must, but take the first step.

Daily Wellness Tracker

Date: _____
S M T W T F S

Today's Fitness Focus

Cardio Strength Flexibility Rest
☐　　　☐　　　　☐　　　　☐

Activity _____
_____

Duration: _____

Today I'm grateful for:

Energy Meter
1 > 2 > 3 > 4 > 5 > 6 > 7 > 8 > 9 > 10

Stress Indicator
Low　　　Ok　　　High

Water
☐ ☐ ☐ ☐ ☐ ☐ ☐ ☐

Fruits & Vegetables
☐ ☐ ☐ ☐ ☐ ☐ ☐ ☐

	Meal Tracker	Counter*
Breakfast		
Lunch		
Dinner		
Snacks		

*Calories, points, containers

Notes

Some Days You Eat Salads And Go To The Gym, Some Days You Eat Cupcakes And Refuse To Put On Pants. It's Called **BALANCE.**

Daily Wellness Tracker

Date: _____
S M T W T F S

Today's Fitness Focus

Cardio ☐   Strength ☐   Flexibility ☐   Rest ☐

Activity _____
_____

Duration: _____

Today I'm grateful for:

Energy Meter
1 > 2 > 3 > 4 > 5 > 6 > 7 > 8 > 9 > 10

Stress Indicator
Low   Ok   High

Water
☐ ☐ ☐ ☐ ☐ ☐ ☐ ☐

Fruits & Vegetables
☐ ☐ ☐ ☐ ☐ ☐ ☐

	Meal Tracker	Counter*
Breakfast		
Lunch		
Dinner		
Snacks		

* Calories, points, containers

Notes

Start
...Do
...Finish

Daily Wellness Tracker

Date: _____
S M T W T F S

Today's Fitness Focus

Cardio ☐   Strength ☐   Flexibility ☐   Rest ☐

Activity _____
_____

Duration: _____

Today I'm grateful for:

Energy Meter
1 > 2 > 3 > 4 > 5 > 6 > 7 > 8 > 9 > 10

Stress Indicator
Low   Ok   High

Water
☐ ☐ ☐ ☐ ☐ ☐ ☐ ☐

Fruits & Vegetables
☐ ☐ ☐ ☐ ☐ ☐ ☐

	Meal Tracker	Counter*
Breakfast		
Lunch		
Dinner		
Snacks		

* Calories, points, containers

Notes

Never Give Up On Your Dreams

Daily Wellness Tracker

Date: _____
S M T W T F S

Today's Fitness Focus

Cardio ☐ Strength ☐ Flexibility ☐ Rest ☐

Activity _____

Duration: _____

Today I'm grateful for:

Energy Meter
1 2 3 4 5 6 7 8 9 10

Stress Indicator
Low Ok High

Water
☐ ☐ ☐ ☐ ☐ ☐ ☐ ☐

Fruits & Vegetables
☐ ☐ ☐ ☐ ☐ ☐ ☐

	Meal Tracker	Counter*
Breakfast		
Lunch		
Dinner		
Snacks		

*Calories, points, containers

Notes

You Are Unstoppable, Go Be Awesome Today!

Daily Wellness Tracker

Date: _____
S M T W T F S

Today's Fitness Focus

Cardio ☐ Strength ☐ Flexibility ☐ Rest ☐

Activity _____

Duration: _____

Today I'm grateful for:

Energy Meter

1 > 2 > 3 > 4 > 5 > 6 > 7 > 8 > 9 > 10

Stress Indicator

Low | Ok | High

Water
☐ ☐ ☐ ☐ ☐ ☐ ☐ ☐

Fruits & Vegetables
☐ ☐ ☐ ☐ ☐ ☐ ☐ ☐

	Meal Tracker	Counter*
Breakfast		
Lunch		
Dinner		
Snacks		

*Calories, points, containers

Notes

Work Hard
Dream Big
Never Give Up

Daily Wellness Tracker

Date: _____
S M T W T F S

Today's Fitness Focus

Cardio Strength Flexibility Rest
☐   ☐   ☐   ☐

Activity _____

_____

Duration: _____

Today I'm grateful for:

Energy Meter

1 2 3 4 5 6 7 8 9 10

Stress Indicator

Low   Ok   High

Water
☐ ☐ ☐ ☐ ☐ ☐ ☐ ☐

Fruits & Vegetables
☐ ☐ ☐ ☐ ☐ ☐ ☐

	Meal Tracker	Counter*
Breakfast		
Lunch		
Dinner		
Snacks		

* Calories, points, containers

Notes

She Believed She Could So She Did

Daily Wellness Tracker

Date: _____
S M T W T F S

Today's Fitness Focus

Cardio Strength Flexibility Rest
☐   ☐   ☐   ☐

Activity _____
_____

Duration: _____

Today I'm grateful for:

Energy Meter
1 > 2 > 3 > 4 > 5 > 6 > 7 > 8 > 9 > 10

Stress Indicator
Low   Ok   High

Water
☐ ☐ ☐ ☐ ☐ ☐ ☐ ☐

Fruits & Vegetables
☐ ☐ ☐ ☐ ☐ ☐ ☐

Meal Tracker | Counter*

	Meal Tracker	Counter*
Breakfast		
Lunch		
Dinner		
Snacks		

* Calories, points, containers

Notes

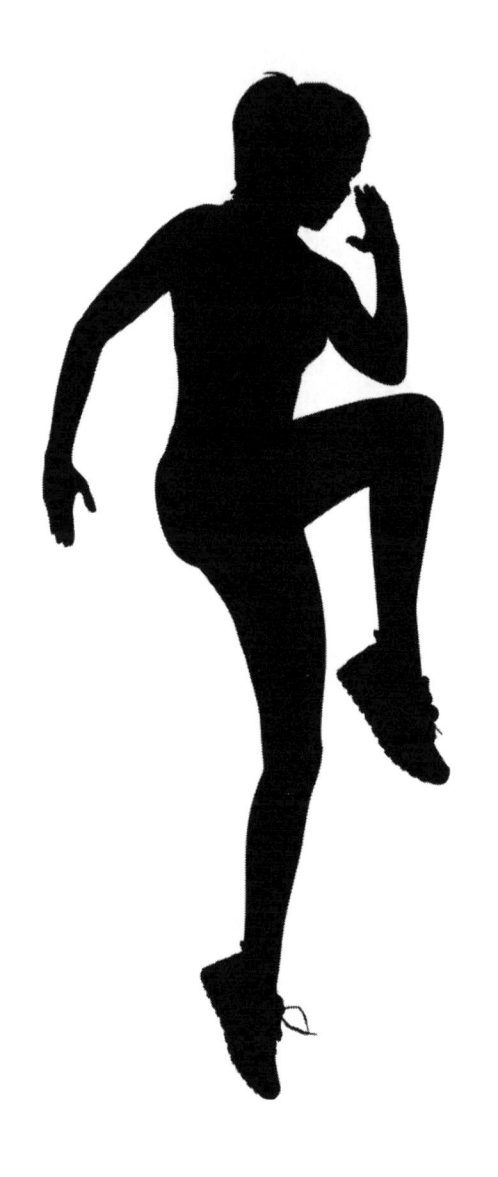

Accomplishments

START WEIGHT:

CURRENT WEIGHT:

TOTAL LOSS:

I can do anything...

MY ACCOMPLISHMENTS:

NOTES TO SELF:

Believe in Yourself

Made in the USA
Columbia, SC
28 January 2022